Table of Contents

Introduction

I would like to begin by explaining why I actually decided to write this book. I hope you have already heard the buzzword "lectins", because that would make my job so much easier. Even if you did, do you really know what lectins are and why they get this much attention today?

Lectin plays an important role in our immune system. It is a type of protein that attaches to the cells in the form of sticky molecules. Lectins can be found in plenty of foods that we eat every day. The most essential sources of lectins are plants, meat, and dairy. But have you ever heard about the negative effect the lectins have on human health? They are difficult to digest and can also bind to the cells in a person's gut, causing different diseases and inflammations. But don't worry, there is some news – despite how scary lectins sound they don't cause much damage when eaten in moderate amounts. I feel like the majority of the readers didn't even know that lectins can be found in the food we consume every day. And it's not like you can avoid these ingredients in your daily life either. One may say that it is impossible to avoid your favorite foods.

However, I'm sure that if you read all the recipes suggested in this book carefully, you will be surprised with a variety of dishes and the combinations of the ingredients included. For those, suffering from symptoms of the leaky gut syndrome or any other terrible digestive disorder, the consumption of lectin-free foods could bring the much needed relief.

Living in a fast-paced world of today, being in a rush all day long seven days per week, nobody wants to spend time searching for the lectin-free recipes. And that's exactly when this book comes to the rescue! All the healthy recipes are structured in separate chapters and are very easy to find. I hope my book will become your best friend in the kitchen!

Chapter 1

What Are Lectins?

A type of the protein that is able to bind to the cell membrane is usually called lectin. Lectins bind to the "glyco," portion of glycoconjugates found on cell membranes and are sugar-binding. They allow species to exist without involving the defense system that might affect the cell-cell interaction. There are a plenty of lectins in grains and raw legumes, in dairy products and some kinds of vegetables. Lectins found in plants protect them against pests, microorganisms and insects; they are resistant to the human digestive system and enter the bloodstream unaltered. So, what happens after the unaltered lectins enter the human body? First of all, they cause severe damage to the intestinal lining that could result in the leaky gut syndrome. And when rough food abounded with lectins is left in the digestive tract for a while it doesn't look very promising. In fact, it looks a lot like the cause behind such autoimmune diseases like MS, Crohn's, fibromyalgia, Hashimoto's, chronic fatigue syndrome, IBS, rheumatoid arthritis… What's more is that lectins are linked with leptin stamina. This is a pre-diabetic condition related to obesity. Leptin, being an essential hormone produced by fat tissue, is responsible for appetite regulation. When the production of this hormone is damaged, it is easy to overeat as the brain gets no message that the stomach is full. The aftermath could lead to an increased glucose level and actually II type diabetes.

For example, a large amount of lectin called „phytohaemagglutinin" can be found in red beans. Perhaps, not everybody has heard about the so-called „red kidney bean poisoning", which is a type of a medical complication that causes nausea, diarrhea and vomiting. This poisoning is a result of consuming undercooked or raw kidney beans. But don't be scared. Remember, we can avoid lectins by boiling the beans while cooking different dishes. Sprouting and soaking can remove all lectins as well. And, I hope nobody prefers eating raw kidney beans anyway.

Is It Safe to Eat Lectins?

Thinking about the question of how safe lectin consumption is, one should remember that the foods high in lectins also contain protein, some essential minerals and vitamins. The lectin is definitely toxic and dangerous in large doses. But, of course, I don't think you sit at home and eat lectins with a spoon! We can avoid consuming too much lectin by simply limiting or properly cooking the ingredients that contain this particular protein. People who have issues with their digestive or immune system are easily able to stick to the lectin-free diet, despite the fact that it is contained in many products we consume every day. In any case, you should remember that a diet must be prescribed by the doctor, so that it doesn't cause any deficiencies of the nutrients essential for the human body.

There are various types of researches conducted to create a list of foods that contain lectins. Those, who aim to avoid or decrease lectin consumption, may find the following list of dietary limitations useful:

Pulses, beans in particular: they are the real origin of lectins. Pinto, soy, kidney, field and string beans – all of them contain lectins. This category also includes green peas, sweet peas, cowpeas, horse grams, lentils, mung beans and soybean sprouts. So if you really love eating beans and can't imagine your life without them, the only thing you can do is cook them thoroughly. Fermentation destroys lectins just as well as cooking, but it doesn't work with all pulses. For example, lectins in French beans aren't completely eliminated during these processes.

Cereals and grains, like wheat germ, corn, barley, rice and all the dishes made from these grains contain lectin. One of the lectin types that aren't properly digested after consumption can be found in wheat germ. This is something all of you, who like bread and pasta, should keep in mind.

 Vegetables and fruits: among the vegetables that contain lectin are potatoes, tomatoes, carrots, zucchini, beets, rhubarb, asparagus, cucumbers, pumpkin, radishes and sweet peppers. Oranges, lemons and grapefruits contain lectin just like blackberries, strawberries, and raspberries. The other fruits particularly high in lectin are grapes, pomegranates, quinces, cherries, bananas, papayas, watermelons, currants, plums and apples. Usually to limit the negative effect, the doctor will recommend you only in-season fruits but in limited quantity. As for those, who stick to the lectin-free diet, fruits aren't recommended for consumption in the first few weeks.

Meat: one simply must avoid eating meat from the corn-fed animals. It is much better to only get specifically grass-fed meat sold in the stores.

Dairy products: cheese, yogurt, butter, cream and conventional milk – all contain lectin. However, clarified butter, also called ghee, is allowed as a part of the lectin-free diet. Speaking about the products made from sheep or goat milk, they are allowed too, as well as some high-fat kinds of cheese.

Sugar: maple syrup, sugar, and agave are strictly forbidden.

Other foods: if you consume nuts or seeds (even if they are dried or roasted) it means you consume also lectin. Hazelnuts, walnuts, peanuts, coconuts, sesame and sunflower seeds – all are a source of lectin. It can also be found in certain spices (like nutmeg, caraway, marjoram, peppermint, etc.), coffee and chocolate.

Having read this long list of products you should stay away from, you surely are thinking so what is safe to eat? Today we have access to a huge variety of products that may easily replace those included in the list of dietary limitations. For those, wishing to reduce their lectin intake the following foods are recommended for consumption:

Green veggies and leafy greens;

Cruciferous vegetables, like Brussels sprouts, broccoli, etc.;

onions;

celery;

avocadoes and mushrooms;

extra virgin olive oil and olives in general;

meat (pasture-raised poultry and beef);

fish;

A-2 milk. Casein A-2 is a type of a protein that can typically be found in dairy products made from goat's, sheep's and Jersey cow's milk. A-1 protein that is found in most cow's milk today may attach to the B cells of the pancreas when being processed by the body and cause an autoimmune attack. There are indeed some people who cannot imagine their lives without milk. I would say that those people should try to drink only organic A-2 milk (raw milk is even better) produced from grass-fed cows.

I'm sure you understand that it is impossible to completely eliminate lectins from one's diet. However, it is a great idea to begin by eliminating the products that are especially high in lectins. Before selecting a diet always consult your doctor and take into account the specifics of your body and your digestive health.

Lectin-Free Meal Plan

I think we all know that at it is not very unusual for people to suddenly decide that it is time to make changes and follow a certain diet. Although, some people are scared of the word „diet", because they think it means they will have to limit all food consumption, just drink water and dream about that medium-rare steak they will be able to eat after the diet is over. Most of us promise ourselves to start eating healthy and clean tomorrow. But tomorrow comes and nothing changes. We repeat the promise again and again. This time should be different, looking through the previously provided information and realizing that you actually want to stick to lectin-free foods, you have to also understand that the best day to begin your diet is today! There is no time to waste, if you look it up you'll see that many researchers have to come to a conclusion that lectin is one of the most harmful food components out there.

So where do you start? First of all, you need to prepare your body. Just like the gardener prepares the soil before he starts planting new fruits and vegetables, in the same way you need to prepare the body for possible future changes that may come with cutting the consumption of high-lectin foods. It might be a little difficult to start the lectin-free diet, but overall, the positive effect will definitely be worth the effort.

The lectin-free diet is well-known for its health-boosting and weight loss benefits. The list of other lectin-free diet advantages includes:

Helping reduce inflammation – lectin-free diet helps to avoid diabetes, celiac disease, rheumatoid arthritis and others autoimmune diseases;

One may increase the chances of avoiding depression, cancer or other serious medical illnesses with the help of the lectin-free diet;

Lectin-free diet improves the balance of the person's gut bacteria;

It helps you shed a few extra pounds;

This type of diet improves your overall well-being.

However, going into this you have to understand that after consuming high-lectin products for such a long time you gut is already damaged even if there haven't been any obvious symptoms yet. If you do decide to stick with the lectin-free diet there are a couple of rules you will need to accept: eating natural foods, cooked products, veggies, avocadoes, mostly white grains, cooking with extra virgin olive oil and removing all peels and seeds from vegetables and fruits before consumption. The lectin-free diet is advantageous and very beneficial but still, it comes with some cons and risks for those, who already have certain health issues and this exactly why you have to consult your doctor before starting this journey.

A Short Lectin-Free Meal Plan

Here is a short lectin-free weekly meal plan thas desired help you get started:

Day 1: Lectin-Free Pancakes / Lectin-Free Coconut Chicken / Creamed Cabbage

Day 2: Lectin-Free Spicy Turmeric Sweet Potato Fries / Green Turkey casserole / Special Tandoori Cauliflower

Day 3: Venison Breakfast Sausage / Almond-Crusted Chicken Strips / Indian Cauliflower "Rice"

Day 4: Lectin-Free Spicy Turmeric Sweet Potato Fries / Shoyu Chicken / Romaine Leaf Caesar Burger Wraps

Day 5: Lectin-Free Bread / Almond-Crusted Chicken Strips / Sweet Potato Hash

Day 6: Parsnip and Spinach Frittata / White Zinfandel Chicken / Healthy Tuna Salad in Avocados

Day 7: Easy Almond Flour Biscuits / Rosemary Roasted Turkey / "Petit Dejeuner" Salad

Breakfasts

Easy Almond Flour Biscuits

These biscuits, containing only five simple ingredients, such as almond flour (that is allowed during your lectin-free diet), an egg, baking powder, ghee, and salt are very light and delicious. They are easy to make and are a great way to start your day! You may cook them using a springform pan if you like.

Ingredients (5 servings):

1 1/2 cup	blanched almond flour
1 tsp	baking powder
1/2 tsp	kosher salt (or ca. 1/4 tsp salt)
3 tbsp	butter (ghee)
1	egg

Directions:

1) First of all, preheat your oven to 350 F and line the bottom of the cookie shit (the springform) with parchment paper to prevent the biscuits sticking to it.

2) Take a medium-sized bowl and add salt, baking powder, and almond flour. Mix well with a spoon.

3) Add ghee to the dry ingredients in the bowl and mix thoroughly until the dough is crumbly. Make sure there are no big lumps in the dough.

4) Make a well in the middle of the dough in the bowl. Take an egg and crack it right into the well. Mix using a fork, slowly incorporating the egg into the dough. Your dough has to be soft.

5) Wash your hands, dry with a paper towel. Divide the dough using your hands into four equal pieces and roll them into balls. You may use a little bit of almond flour so that the dough doesn't stick to your hands.

6) Take the lined cookie sheet and put the balls onto it. Try to not flatten them out. Bake the biscuits for about 25 minutes until they are golden.

7) After 25 minutes take the cookie sheet out of the oven, remove the biscuits and serve. Let them cool a little before eating.

Bon Appetite!

Lectin-free Bread

This recipe for lectin-free, flavorful and soft bread is simple and delicious! You may add your favorite spices to this recipe, depending on your mood and the preferences of the people you will share it with. I usually add some Italian seasonings and eat it both for breakfast and dinner. It is a perfect addition to meat, fish and green salads!

Ingredients (7 servings):

3/4 cup	ghee
4	eggs, beaten
1/3 cup	almond flour
1 tsp	baking powder
1/2 tsp	kosher salt
1 tsp	sweetener of choice
1 tsp	herbs of choice (optional)

Directions:

1) Preheat your oven to 350F.

2) Take a loaf pan of your choice (depending on what shape of bread you want). Line your form with parchment paper, if you are using a silicone form you can skip this step.

3) Take a little pot and heat the ghee in it.

4) Take a bigger bowl and add the heated ghee, baking powder, salt, almond flour, sweetener of your choice and mix well. Add the eggs to the mixture and continue stirring until homogenous. Make sure that there are no lumps in the mix. Add the preferred herbs.

5) Once the dough is ready, pour it into the prepared loaf pan. When pouring the dough do not fill the form up to the brim, leave some space for the dough to rise.

6) Put the bread in the oven and let it bake for 45 minutes. Avoid opening the oven often to check on the bread otherwise it may fail to rise properly.

7) After 45 minutes (using a toothpick make sure that the center of the loaf is set), turn off the oven and leave the bread in for a few more minutes. Remove it from the oven and let it cool.

8) Slice on the cutting board and serve.

Bon Appetite!

Parsnip and Spinach Frittata

It seems to me that we all like to start our days with something quick and easy but filling and nutritious. That's why I would like to recommend you my healthy parsnip and spinach frittata. It takes 40 minutes to make it, but 35 of them your oven will do the work for you. And you can just get ready in the meantime.

Ingredients (5 servings):

4	whole eggs
2 tsp	olive oil
1 pce	large parsnip
1 cup	spinach
1/4 tsp	herbs

Directions:

1)   Preheat the oven to 350F.

2) Take a large parsnip, wash it thoroughly, peel and chop into cubes.

3) Wash the spinach, dry it with a paper towel. Chop it up if it is large. Set aside.

4) Take a medium-sized skillet, heat the skillet and add olive oil.

5) Add parsnips into the skillet and cook for about 10 minutes until they become golden brown. Then add chopped (or whole) spinach.

6) Take fresh eggs and crack them over the vegetables into the skillet. Stir the eggs into the vegetables.

7) Sprinkle with salt and herbs as desired. Add black pepper. Bake everything in the oven for about 35 minutes until the top becomes golden brown. Check on the frittata from time to time, as it could be ready sooner.

8) Once the time is over, take the frittata out the oven and put it onto a large plate. Slice to serve. Eat while still hot.

Bon Appetite!

Lectin-Free Spicy Turmeric Sweet Potato Fries

These spicy turmeric sweet potato fries are easy and quick to make. It is just like making fries from regular potatoes. Add your favorite herbs while baking the fries and you get delicious crispy potato slices for breakfast. Both adults and kids enjoy this lectin-free dish!

Ingredients (6 servings):

1	large sweet potato
1 tablespoon	100% pure avocado oil

For the seasoning:

1/2 teaspoon	turmeric powder
1/2 teaspoon	cayenne pepper
1/2 teaspoon	ground black pepper
1/2 teaspoon	pink salt

Directions:

1) Firstly, preheat the oven to 425F.

2) Wash and peel the sweet potato. Slice it into long pieces the „French fry" style. If you have a large sweet potato you should get around 50 pieces or less.

3) Once the sweet potato is cut, put it into a large bowl. Pour the avocado oil over the slices and toss everything well. Make sure all of the slices are well-coated.

4) Add turmeric, cayenne pepper, black pepper and pink salt to the mixing bowl with the sweet potato slices. Mix everything using your hands.

5) Put some parchment paper on the base of the baking tray where you plan to bake your fries.

6) Put the sweet potato pieces onto a baking tray and bake at 425 degrees for 20 minutes.

7) After 20 minutes, take the tray out of the oven, flip your fries and put them back in the oven for a few more minutes. It should take 10 minutes maximum. The fries when done must be crispy and golden brown.

Enjoy while still hot!

Venison Breakfast Sausage

It doesn't take a lot of time to make these venison breakfast sausages and what's even better is that they can be made beforehand and stored in the fridge. Everything you need to do right before breakfast is heat the skillet and fry the sausages over the high heat. They are juicy, flavorful and light. You can spice them up a bit by adding a little bit of minced onion.

Ingredients (9 servings):

1 pound	ground venison
8 ounces	bacon
1 teaspoon	ground sage
1/2 teaspoon	ground ginger
1/4 teaspoon	pepper
3/4 teaspoon	onion salt
1	egg
½ cup	almond flour
3 tsp	olive oil

Directions:

1) Take a large mixing bowl, add the ground venison.

2) Cut the bacon strips into small bits and add the bacon to the ground venison. Toss everything well.

3) Add ground sage, salt, pepper and ground ginger. Crack the egg into your meat mixture. Stir everything well until smooth.

4) Using your hands (wet them with some tap water) shape the mixture into same-size patties (or long sausages if you'd like).

5) Take a little plate or a cutting board. Sprinkle with almond flour. Roll the patties (sausages) in the almond flower.

6) Take a medium-sized skillet, heat the skillet and add some olive oil.

7) Once the oil is hot, place the sausages onto the skillet and fry on all sides, 3-5 minutes per each side.

8) Take the cooked sausages off the heat and serve.

Enjoy hot!

Bon Appetite!

Lectin-Free Pancakes

If you love pancakes and can't imagine your breakfast without them – this recipe is for you! There are definitely many different pancake recipes you have already tried. My recipe, however, is special as it is lectin-free and therefore suitable for the lectin-free diet.

Ingredients (6 servings):

4	large omega-3 eggs
2 teaspoons	pure vanilla extract
4 - 5 tablespoons	extra-virgin coconut oil
1⁄4 cup	sweetener
1⁄8 teaspoon	sea salt
1⁄2 teaspoon	baking soda

Directions:

1) Take a medium-sized bowl, crack fresh eggs into it. Beat them with a blender until smooth.

2) Add vanilla extract to the egg mix. Melt the coconut oil and add into the bowl.

3) Add sweetener, salt and baking soda. Mix until smooth for about 3-4 minutes.

4) Take a small pan, add coconut oil and heat the pan over medium-high heat. Once the oil begins to bubble, take a cup and fill ½ of it with batter. Pour the batter onto the pan, spread well. Once one side of the pancake is golden brown, flip it over and wait for a few more minutes (2-3).

5) When the bottom side of the pancake is done, the top will look fairly dry with a few bubbles on top.

6) Don't forget to add oil to the bottom of the pan if needed for the new pancakes. You may use the silicone cooking brush to spread the oil easily over the bottom of the pan.

Serve hot!

Bon Appetite!

Poultry Dishes

Rosemary Roasted Lectin-Free Turkey

Preparing the meat or fish usually takes us a lot of time. Today I would like to share with you a quick and easy recipe for a delicious whole turkey cooked in a rosemary-basil mix. I like to add the Italian seasoning to mine, but any other herbs of your choice would also work well.

Ingredients (5 servings):

3/4 cup	olive oil
2 tablespoons	fresh rosemary
1 tablespoon	fresh basil
1 tablespoon	Italian seasoning
salt to taste	
1 (12 pounds)	whole turkey

Directions:

1) Before cooking the turkey you must preheat the oven to 350F.

2) Wash and chop fresh rosemary and basil.

3) Take a small bowl, add the olive oil, salt, Italian seasoning, basil, and rosemary. Mix well and set aside.

4) Wash the turkey thoroughly (inside and out) and dry with a paper towel. Remove the skin from the breasts by pulling it slowly with your fingers.

5) Take the herb mixture and spread it all over the turkey (breasts, drumsticks, thighs) and in the cavity using your hands.

6) Take a large roasting pan and add about ¼ inch of water to it. Place your turkey into the pan and put it in the over for 3-4 hours.

7) After a half an hour open the oven and using a spoon pour the liquid (from the bottom of the roasting pan) over the top of the turkey. If you have a cooking thermometer, check the temperature of the meat from time to time. The internal temperature must reach 180F.

8) Once the turkey is ready (check it with the knife or with the thermometer), turn off the oven, but allow the turkey to rest there for a few more minutes.

9) Remove the turkey onto a large tray and carve. Serve with hot sauces and fresh vegetables.

Bon Appetite!

White Zinfandel Chicken

This chicken is super soft and flavorful. The wine gives it a special taste and tenderness and a mix of spices – a delicate aroma. The meat goes great in combination with leafy greens, lectin-free bread, and sauces of choice. You may store the cooked breasts in the fridge for 4-5 days.

Ingredients (7 servings):

2-4 pcs	chicken breast halves
2 teaspoons	avocado oil
1/2 teaspoon	dried rosemary
1/2 teaspoon	dried basil
1/2 teaspoon	dried thyme
1 tablespoon	olive oil
1/2 cup	white Zinfandel wine

Directions:

1) Wash the chicken breasts. Dry with a paper towel. Remove the skin and bones from the breasts. Place the chicken breasts into a medium-sized bowl.

2) In another small bowl combine avocado oil, dried basil and rosemary, dried thyme, pepper and salt. Stir everything well. Pour this mixture over the chicken breasts, use your hands to thoroughly spread it and leave for a half an hour to rest.

3) Take a large skillet, add olive oil and heat it over the medium heat. Once the oil begins to bubble put the chicken breasts onto the skillet. Cook them for 5-6 minutes on one side, flip over and continue cooking. Wait until they become golden brown and a little crispy.

4) Pour the wine into the skillet with the chicken. Check the heat – it must be not higher than medium. Let the alcohol evaporate.

5) Once the chicken breasts are golden brown check them for readiness using a fork or a knife to pierce the breasts. If the juice is clear and the breasts are soft, they are ready.

7) Remove the chicken breasts onto a cutting board and slice while they are still hot.

Bon Appetite!

Almond-Crusted Chicken Strips

These crusted chicken strips are easy to make and are a great treat for the parties, as well as for quiet family dinners. Kids like them very much because they are crispy just like French fries. But if you cook the chicken strips for kids, don't use hot paprika, salt and almond meal will work just fine.

Ingredients (5 servings):

1 lb	chicken breasts
1 cup	almond meal
1 Tbsp	paprika
1 tsp	Himalayan salt
2	eggs (lightly beaten)

Directions:

1) Preheat the oven to 350F.

2) Wash the chicken breasts. Dry with a paper towel. Remove the skin and bones from the breasts. Slice them into long strips of equal size, approximately 1-2 inches wide. Place the chicken strips into a medium-sized bowl.

3) Take another medium-sized bowl and combine salt, paprika and almond meal.

4) Crack fresh eggs into a different bowl and beat them slightly.

5) Take a large baking tray and sprinkle it with olive oil or cooking spray.

6) Take a chicken strip and place it first into the egg mixture and then into the almond meal coating. It must be well-coated from all the sides.

7) Put the chicken strips onto a baking tray, leaving gaps between the strips to prevent them from sticking to each other.

8) Bake them for 25 minutes in the oven. After 5-10 minutes take the tray out and flip the strips.

9) Remove cooked chicken strips from the oven and serve.

Enjoy with hot sauce or ketchup!

Bon Appetite!

Lectin-Free Shoyu Chicken

I think there is no need to wait until these chicken thighs will cool down. They are so flavorful and delicious that one may eat all of them just as soon as they are ready and still hot! Garnish the plate of shoyu chicken with fresh parsley or other herbs of choice and you've got yourself a perfect poultry dish.

Ingredients (9 servings):

1 cup	soy sauce
1 cup	sweetener
1 cup	water
1 tbsp	grated fresh ginger root
1 tbsp	ground black pepper
1 tbsp	dried oregano
1 tbsp	ground cayenne pepper (as desired)
1 Tsp	ground paprika (as desired)
5 pounds	skinless chicken thighs

Fresh parsley for garnish.

Directions:

1) Peel and grate the fresh ginger root.

2) Wash and chop fresh parsley. Set aside.

3) Take a medium-sized bowl, add sweetener, soy sauce, ginger, water, pepper, oregano, cayenne pepper and paprika. Combine everything well and set aside.

4) Wash the chicken thighs thoroughly and dry them with a paper towel. Put them into a large bowl.

5) Pour the mix over the chicken thighs, toss and cover. Put the bowl into the refrigerator for an hour or more. You may leave them in the fridge overnight and cook early in the morning.

6) Take a large frying pan, add a little bit of olive oil, about 2-3 spoons. Don't add more as you will also add the marinade from the chicken to the pan.

7) Heat the frying pan and wait until oil begins to bubble. Carefully take the chicken thighs from the marinade and put them onto the pan. Roast for a few minutes per side, turn from time to time. It usually takes 10-12 minutes per side.

8) Remove the cooked chicken thighs into the plate, dress with freshly chopped parsley and eat immediately.

Bon Appetite!

Lectin-Free Coconut Chicken

Lectin-free chicken with coconut and parsley is a great crowd-pleaser! Serve this flavorful dish with fresh veggies and tasty sauces! Don't hesitate and make this fantastic dish today!

Ingredients (4 servings):

1 (5–6 lb)   whole chicken

1/2 tsp   Himalayan salt

½ cup   coconut oil

4 Tbsp   Italian flat-leaf parsley

Pepper if desired

Directions:

1) Preheat the oven to 350F.

2) Wash the chicken thoroughly and dry with a paper towel. Remove all the insides. Season it finely with salt.

3) Take a large baking dish and place the chicken in the center. The baking dish must not be shallow, so that you could use the liquid from the bottom of the dish and pour it over the chicken as it is baking.

4) Season the chicken with pepper. Place the baking dish with chicken into the oven for 3-4 hours depending on the size of the chicken.

5) After an hour open the oven, gather the liquid carefully from the bottom of the dish (use a spoon and a cup) and pour over the chicken. Do it every 30 minutes.

6) Wash and chop fresh parsley.

7) Take a small bowl, combine parsley and coconut oil. Heat it until the coconut oil melts.

8) When the cooking time is almost over open the oven, pour the oil mixture over the chicken and let it cook for a few more minutes in the oven.

9) Take the chicken out of the oven and serve!

Bon Appetite!

Green Turkey Casserole

Green turkey casserole is an amazing and flavorful dish that I usually cook for supper for my friends and family. It is simple and quick! Try making it yourself!

Ingredients (3 servings):

1 pound	spinach, rinsed and chopped
1 1/2 cups	cooked turkey
2	fresh eggs

Salt and pepper if desired

Parsley for garnish

Directions:

1) Take a medium-sized pot, cook the turkey breasts. Once ready, remove from the pot and let them cool. Cut into cubes.

2) Preheat the oven to 350 degrees F. Prepare one 10-inch casserole dish.

3) Wash the spinach thoroughly and chop finely.

4) Take the casserole dish, spray it with cooking spray or sprinkle with olive oil to prevent burning at the bottom.

5) Place the spinach onto the bottom of the casserole dish. Put the cubed meat over the spinach. Sprinkle with pepper and salt.

6) Take the fresh eggs and crack them into a little bowl. Whisk the eggs finely together. Pour the egg mixture over the other ingredients in the casserole dish.

7) Place the casserole dish into the oven and bake for 20-30 minutes. From time to time check if ready.

Remove from the oven and enjoy while hot!

Bon Appetite!

Seafood Dishes

Crusted Seared Ahi Tuna Appetizer Bites

These wonderful and tender tuna bites couldn't be left without attention. This is a great party appetizer that all of your guests will enjoy. It doesn't take very long to cook, just about a half an hour or so. If you don't like hot spices, don't use sriracha (as it is optional) or chives.

Ingredients (7 servings):

1 pce (about ½ pound)   tuna steak

1 tbsp   tamari or coconut aminos

a dash sriracha (optional)

2 tsp   fresh ginger

2 stalks   chives

3 tbsp   almond flour

3 tbsp   olive oil

Pepper and salt as desired

Cilantro for garnish

Directions:

1) Take the fresh ginger and grate it.

2) Thinly slice the chives.

3) Rinse the tuna steaks, slice them into 1 1/2 inch cubes.

4) Take a medium-sized plate, add almond flour and a little bit of pepper and salt. Roll the tuna pieces in the mixture to coat all sides well. Set aside.

5) Take a pan and place it over medium heat. Sprinkle olive oil over the bottom of the pan and spread it.

6) Once the oil begins to bubble, place the tuna pieces onto the bottom of the pan, and cook for 30 seconds per side until the crust is lightly browned on each side. Be careful and don't burn the fish.

7) Remove tuna pieces from the pan and let them cool. Cut each piece into smaller slices, about 3 medium slices per cube. Arrange them on a serving plate.

8) Take a small bowl and prepare the dressing for the fish. Add sriracha, tamari, grated ginger and a little bit of oil. Whisk everything well until smooth.

9) Sprinkle over tuna bites, top with chives and fresh cilantro.

Enjoy warm!

Bon Appetite!

Roasted Sardines with Herb Crust

What could be quicker and easier than to prepare roasted sardines in the oven? You don't need to stay near the skillet and check with a fork if the fish is ready. Just place it in the oven and when you feel the delicious aroma it means, the sardines are ready!

Ingredients (7 servings):

1 pound	fresh sardines
2 tsp	French mustard
1 Tbsp	dry oregano
½ tsp	paprika
¼ tsp	salt
3 Tbsp	olive oil
2 tsp	fresh parsley

Directions:

1) Firstly, preheat the oven to 425 F.

2) Clean the sardines. Rinse them and dry with a paper towel.

3) Wash and chop fresh parsley.

4) Take a large mixing bowl, add mustard, oregano, paprika, salt and olive oil. Mix everything well.

5) Add the sardines to the mixture and coat them gently until evenly coated.

6) Take a large baking tray and sprinkle with olive oil. Place the sardines onto the tray. They must be in one layer but not too close to each other. Drizzle the rest of the dressing over the fish.

7) Place the tray into the oven and roast for 20 minutes. Flip the fish from time to time checking the readiness.

8) Remove the tray from the oven after 20 minutes. Put them onto a large plate and dress with freshly chopped parsley.

Bon Appetite!

Simple Lectin-Free Garlic Shrimp

Delicious, tender and simply amazing shrimp! If you haven't made or tried this recipe before, don't hesitate to make it today! Minced garlic and pepper give the shrimp a soft kick and the thick sauce makes it incredibly tender.

Ingredients (7 servings):

1 1/2 tsp	olive oil
1 pound	shrimp
6 cloves	garlic
1/4 tsp	red pepper flakes
1 1/2 tsp	ghee
1/3 cup	fresh parsley
1 1/2 Tbsp	broth

Salt to taste

Directions:

1) Peel and wash the shrimps.

2) Peel garlic cloves and mince them finely.

3) Take a skillet and place it over medium heat, wait until oil begins to simmer. Place the shrimp in one layer onto the bottom of the skillet. Cook for about 1 minute. Do not stir. Sprinkle with salt. Continue cooking until shrimp get the pink color. It will take approximately 1-2 minutes more.

4) Add minced garlic and red pepper flakes. Cook for about 1-2 minutes. Add ghee. Add a half of the parsley. Cook until ghee is fully melted.

5) Turn heat to low and add broth. Toss until ghee is fully melted and a thick sauce forms. It takes around 3 minutes.

6) Remove the shrimp from the skillet and place the prepared shrimp into a medium-sized bowl, but continue cooking the sauce. Add one teaspoon of water or broth if the sauce is too thick. Add pepper and salt as desired.

7) Serve shrimp on a plate and dress with hot sauce. Dress finely with the rest of the parsley.

Bon Appetite!

Tender Lectin-Free Mussels

Everything you need to know about these mussels is that they only take 4-5 minutes to cook. However, it is crucial to not overcook the mussels, because that would spoil the whole dish. A particularly flavorful and tender broth will be a great so-called «base» for the mussels.

Ingredients (6 servings):

4 quarts	mussels
6 tablespoons	chopped fresh parsley
1 pce	bay leaf
1/4 teaspoon	dried thyme
2 cups	white wine
3 tablespoon	olive oil

Pepper and salt to taste

Directions:

1) Clean and scrub mussels. Pull the "beards", the seaweed attached to the shell and chop them off with a special paring knife at the base. Set aside.

2) Wash and chop fresh parsley. Set aside.

3) Take a medium-sized mixing bowl. Add parsley, thyme and bay leaf. Add wine and combine everything well.

4) Take a pot and place it over the medium heat. Pour olive oil into the pot and ass the mixture from the mixing bowl. Wait until it begins to boil.

5) Turn the heat to low. Cook the mix about 2-3 minutes.

6) Add cleaned mussels and cover the pot.

7) Cook them until they open, not any longer. It usually takes up to 5 minutes. Check often as the mussels mustn't be overcooked.

8) Take the mussels out of the pot, put them on large plate and dress with rest of fresh parsley.

Bon Appetite!

Ginger Glazed Mahi Mahi

This glazed Mahi Mahi is super crispy, tender and delicious. It takes just a little bit of time and effort to cook it in a large skillet. Grated ginger root adds a special taste to the fish.

Ingredients (7 servings):

1 tbsp	sweetener
3 tbsp	soy sauce
3 tbsp	balsamic vinegar
1 tsp	ginger root
2 tsp	olive oil
4 (6 ounces)	Mahi Mahi fillets

Salt as desired

Pepper optional

1 tbsp	vegetable oil

Directions:

1) Grate ginger root. Set aside.

2) Take a small bowl, add sweetener and soy sauce and whisk. Add balsamic vinegar and ginger. Mix well and add olive oil.

3) Wash fillets well and cut carefully. If the fillets have skin on them do not take it off.

4) Sprinkle the fish with some salt. Add pepper. Place the fillets into a bowl and refrigerate for a half an hour or more.

5) Take a large skillet, put it over medium heat and add oil to the skillet. Wait until it starts to simmer.

6) Take the fillets out of the refrigerator. Leave the marinade in a bowl. Fry the fillets on each side until crispy, flip the pieces with a fork once they are tender.

7) Once the fish fillets are ready, put them onto a large serving plate. Keep warm.

8) Take the fillet marinade, pour it into the skillet and heat over the medium heat. Stir until the marinade becomes thick and smooth.

9) Once the marinade sauce is ready, pour it over the fish.

10) Serve immediately after sprinkling with parsley and pepper.

Bon Appetite!

Steelhead Trout Bake with Dijon Mustard

It seems like the trout indeed is one of the most popular fish amongst the seafood-loving families. Its special tenderness and taste are worth noticing, since this fish is also full of minerals and vitamins. It doesn't have too many bones, so the cooking process is very quick and easy.

Ingredients (4 servings):

cooking spray (optional)

1 pound	trout fillets
1/4 cup	dry white wine
2 1/2 tablespoons	Dijon mustard
1 teaspoon	fresh dill

Pepper and salt as desired

Directions:

1) Preheat the oven to 425 degrees F.

2) Take a medium-sized baking dish. Spray it with cooking spray or add a little bit of olive or vegetable oil.

3) Wash and cut the trout fillets. Place them on the baking dish in one layer.

4) Wash and cut fresh dill.

5) Take a small bowl, add dry wine, dill and Dijon mustard. Mix everything well. Pour the mix over the fish.

6) Place the baking dish into the preheated oven. Bake fillets for about 20- 25 minutes or more if the pieces are thick. Make sure the sauce doesn't burn.

7) Once the baking time is over, take the baking dish out of the oven. Sprinkle the fish with pepper and salt if desired.

8) Serve in a baking dish.

Bon Appetite!

Beef Dishes

Spicy-Mustard Glazed Pork Ribs

These spicy-mustard ribs are simply amazing, especially when cooked over a grill. They are crispy on the outside, but tender, flavorful and juicy on the inside! This dish will become the star of your meal on a hot summer day when there are plenty of vegetables that you can combine it with.

Ingredients (7 servings):

2 tbsp	vegetable oil
1 1/2 cups	sweetener
1 cup	Dijon mustard
1/2 cup	cider vinegar
1 tsp	Cajun seasoning
1/2 tsp	salt
2 pounds	pork ribs

pepper as desired

Directions:

1) Before preparing the pork ribs you must preheat the grill to a medium heat.

2) Take a little saucepan and heat the oil over high heat. Add the sweetener and stir constantly. Add mustard and stir again. Carefully pour in the vinegar. Continue stirring.

3) Season the mixture in the saucepan with Cajun seasoning, pepper, and salt as desired. Reduce the heat. Let it simmer for 4 minutes or longer. Once the time is over, take the saucepan of the heat and set aside.

4) Wash the ribs, rinse them well. Dry them with a paper towel. Sprinkle with black pepper and salt to taste, place the pork ribs onto the grill rack. Cover and cook for 20 minutes. After 20 minutes flip the ribs and continue cooking. Don't overcook the ribs but check the readiness from time to time.

5) When the ribs are almost ready, pour the sauce from the saucepan over them and cover for 10-15 minutes.

6) After 15 minutes uncover and transfer the cooked ribs onto a large plate. Dress them with fresh dill or cilantro.

Bon Appetite!

Korean Sesame Beef Lettuce Wraps

This time I offer you to try my super spicy and tender Korean lettuce wraps. I have tried this dish in a restaurant a few years ago and fell in love. Since then I have tried to cook it at home and you won't believe how easy the process is!

Ingredients (7 servings):

3/4 pound	flank steak
2 tablespoons	low-sodium soy sauce
1 teaspoon	olive oil
2 tablespoons	avocado oil
4 cups	cooked cauliflower rice
1 cup	kimchi
16 leaves	lettuce leaves

Directions:

1) Wash the steaks and dry them with a paper towel.

2) Slice the steak into long strips.

3) Take a medium-sized bowl, place the steak strips, add olive oil and soy sauce. Using your hands toss everything well. Set aside.

4) Take a large skillet and place it over medium heat. Add a little bit of avocado oil, wait until it begins to simmer.

5) Once it heats up, add a half of the steak strips into the skillet. Roast until lightly golden brown. It usually takes 2-3 minutes.

6) Take a long spoon and use it to transfer the cooked steak pieces from the skillet into a large bowl.

7) Continue the same procedure with the rest of the steak mix.

8) Take a large plate, take a lettuce leaf, spoon cauliflower rice onto the leaf, add steak strips, add kimchi and roll up. Do the same with all the leaves.

Bon Appetite!

Cream Lectin-Free Chip Beef

This beef is amazing! The onions and cream cheese added to the beef in the cooking process give it a special tenderness. But, while buying groceries to make this dish, don't forget about your lectin-free diet and choose the cream cheese that is produced from A-2 milk only. Read the ingredients on the package carefully!

Ingredients (5 servings):

1 tablespoon	ghee
2.5ounces	beef
4 ounces	Cream Cheese (made from A 2 milk)
1pinch	white pepper
1 pce	white onion

Salt as desired

Directions:

1) Take the beef and rinse it well.

2) Place the beef on the cutting board, dry with a paper towel and chop. Cut it as you wish. I usually cut mine into small pieces as they cook faster. But long strips are also OK.

3) Take a medium-sized skillet and place it over high heat. Add the ghee and wait until it is almost fully melted.

4) Add chopped beef pieces and stir well. Roast them for 5 minutes on one side and slip over.

5) Peel and slice the onions.

6) Roast the beef strips for 5 minutes after flipping. When the pieces are almost ready and tender, add chopped onions and cook them until golden brown.

7) Carefully add cream cheese when both meat and onion are tender. Wait until it melts. Cover, reduce the heat to low and let it cook for 5 minutes. The sauce must become smooth.

8) Remove the skillet from the heat, transfer the beef onto a large bowl. Serve!

Bon Appetite!

Romaine Leaf Caesar Burgers Wraps

I don't know a single person who doesn't like burgers. But what I do know is how to cook lectin-free burgers at home. They are amazing! I personally prefer the burgers without buns, just patties and lettuce. You should try them!

Ingredients (6 servings):

1 1/2 pounds	ground beef
1/4 cup	almond flour
1/2 tsp	poultry seasoning
1/2 cup	Caesar dressing
1/2 teaspoon	black pepper
6 leaves	romaine lettuce
3 tbsp	olive oil

Directions:

1) Preheat the grill to medium heat.

2) Take a medium-sized bowl, add ground beef, seasoning, almond flour, Caesar dressing, pepper and salt. Mix everything well using your hands.

3) Take a little plate and sprinkle it with some flour.

4) Form the burgers by hand and thoroughly coat them with flour.

5) Take a medium-sized skillet and heat the olive oil. Let it simmer a little bit. Place the burgers onto the skillet and roast for 5-6 minutes per side. They must be a little bit crispy.

6) Take a large plate. Place the lettuce leaves over the plate, put the cooked burgers onto the leaves.

7) Top the burgers with the remaining Caesar dressing. Serve hot!

Bon Appetite!

Mediterranean Meatballs

Lectin-free Mediterranean meatballs are easy to prepare for dinner and supper. You may store them in the fridge for a few days and make some hot and spicy sauce to go with your meatballs. Don't hesitate and cook them today!

Ingredients (8 servings):

1 lb	ground beef
¼ cup	almond flour
1 tsp	Italian seasoning
1	large egg
2 Tbsp	fresh parsley
½ tsp	ground cumin
½ tsp	Himalayan salt
¼ tsp	black pepper

Directions:

1) Preheat the oven to 425°F.

2) Take a large bowl, combine ground beef, Italian seasoning, ground cumin and flour. Crack a fresh egg into the mixture. Mix everything well. Season with pepper and salt.

3) Using your hands, form small meatballs and cover in almond flour.

4) Take a large baking sheet, cover it with a parchment paper, put the meatballs on it and place in the oven.

5) Bake them for about 40 minutes, open the oven and check if the meatballs are ready from time to time. They must not be pink on the inside. Remember that the cooking time might depend on the size of the meatballs.

6) Remove the meatballs onto a plate and garnish with fresh parsley and veggies.

Bon Appetite!

Italian Meatballs

These Italian meatballs cooked in the special onion and cream cheese (A-2 milk) sauce are super tender and tasty! The meatballs get the special flavor of fresh chopped parsley and cilantro as well as garlic and onions.

Ingredients (12 servings):

2 lb	ground pork
1 lb	ground beef
2 Tbsp	fresh cilantro
1	egg
1 Tbsp	parsley
2 tsp	kosher salt
1 tsp	black pepper
4 ounces	Cream Cheese (made from A 2 milk)
3 tbsp	almond flour
1	onion
½ tsp	dried garlic
2 tbsp	olive oil

Directions:

1) Preheat the oven to 425 degrees F.

2) Take a mixing bowl, add ground beef, ground pork, salt and pepper. Mix everything well.

3) Wash and chop fresh parsley and cilantro finely. Set aside.

4) Crack the egg and add it to the mixture. Add almond flour.

5) Using your hand roll the meatballs covering them in almond flour.

6) Cover the baking sheet with parchment paper and place the meatballs on top. Place the baking sheet into the oven and bake for 20-25 minutes.

7) While the meatballs are cooking prepare the sauce.

8) Peel the onion and chop it finely. Take a little skillet, add olive oil and wait until it simmers. Add onion and roast until lightly golden.

9) Add dried garlic and cream cheese. Stir everything well. Cook for 5 minutes. Remove the sauce into the medium-sized pot and place over low heat.

10) Once the meatballs are ready, take them from the baking sheet and carefully transfer into the pot with the sauce.

11) Cook for 15 minutes over low heat.

Serve warm!

Bon Appetite!

Vegetable Dishes

Creamed Cabbage

Creamed cabbage is a great side dish to spicy beef or pork. This cabbage is super tender thanks to coconut oil and a cup of A-2 milk added to the skillet. Try adding your favorite spices at the end.

Ingredients (7 servings):

2 Tbsp	coconut oil
1½ lbs	green cabbage
¾ tsp	kosher salt
¼ tsp	black pepper
¼ cup	water, more as needed
1 handful	fresh parsley leaves, for garnish (optional)
1 cup	A-2 milk

Directions:

1) Take a large, deep skillet and add coconut oil. Heat the oil, placing the skillet over medium heat.

2) Take one head of cabbage and slice it finely. Set aside.

3) Once the oil is melted, add cabbage and salt. Mix well. Add pepper, water and cook everything for about 12 minutes.

4) Stir from time to time. Add the water if the there is no liquid on the bottom of the skillet. Check if the cabbage is tender.

5) When the cabbage is tender, add A-2 milk and toss everything well.

6) Stir everything once more and remove from heat.

7) Transfer to a large serving dish.

8) Wash fresh parsley leaves and let them dry. Dress your cabbage with parsley. Sprinkle with black pepper as desired.

Bon Appetite!

Special Tandoori Cauliflower

This cauliflower recipe is easy and quick to make. Everything you need to do is just mix and bake 5 simple ingredients for about half an hour. And just like that your breakfast or a light supper is ready!

Ingredients (5 servings):

3/4 cup	lectin-free cream cheese
2 teaspoons	Tandoori Spice Blend
1 teaspoon	fresh ginger
1/2 teaspoon	kosher salt
1 head (about 1 1/2 lb.)	cauliflower

Directions:

1) Before cooking the cauliflower, preheat the oven to 425F.

2) Peel and grate fresh ginger. Set aside.

3) Wash one medium head of cauliflower.

4) Take a medium-sized bowl, add cream cheese, Tandoori spice, grated ginger and salt. Mix everything well. Add pepper as desired.

5) Take a large baking sheet and spray it with some cooking spray or a little bit of olive oil. Place the cauliflower onto the sheet leaving a little space between the small heads.

6) Put the sheet into the oven and bake for 20 minutes.

7) Once the cooking time is over remove the sheet from the oven and transfer the cauliflower onto the plate. Sprinkle with pepper if desired.

Bon Appetite!

Indian Cauliflower "Rice"

Rice is of the menu during the lectin-free diet. But don't worry, because you can just make this special tasty cauliflower rice that is full of vitamins and minerals. You may serve it as a side dish with fish or meat.

Ingredients (10 servings):

1 head	cauliflower
2 Tbsp	coconut oil
¼ tsp	turmeric
¼ tsp	ground ginger
⅛ tsp	cardamom
⅛ tsp	cinnamon
⅛ tsp	ground cloves
½ tsp	salt
1-2 Tbsp	vegetable oil
3-4 Tbsp	cilantro, to garnish

black pepper as desired

Directions:

1) Take the cauliflower and chop it finely. The florets must be small, approximately 1-2-inches.

2) Using the food processor blend the cauliflower until the florets turn into small rice-sized bits. Set aside.

3) Take a large pan, add the coconut oil and heat it over medium heat. When the oil is melted and starts to simmer, add the cauliflower rice from the food processor. Cook it for about 5-7 minutes.

4) Add turmeric, ground ginger grated, cardamom, cinnamon and ground cloves. Add salt and pepper as desired.

5) Wash and chop fresh cilantro.

6) Remove cauliflower rice from the heat and taste if it is ready.

7) Cover the rice and cook for a few more minutes.

8) Remove the rice onto a plate, dress with cilantro or other spices of your choice.

Bon Appetite!

Sweet Potato Hash

This easy recipe of sweet potato hash with lots of spices is a perfect addition to bacon strips and scrambled eggs for a great breakfast. Serve it immediately after baking!

Ingredients (8 servings):

2 medium	sweet potatoes
2 tbsp	olive or avocado oil
1 tsp	smoked paprika
½ tsp	turmeric
½ tsp	sea salt
½ tsp	onion powder
¼-1/2 tsp	ground black pepper
2 cloves	garlic

Bacon strips for garnish

Directions:

1) Preheat oven to 425 degrees F.

2) Peel and cube the sweet potatoes.

3) Peel and finely mince garlic.

4) Take a medium bowl, add cubed potatoes and oil. Mix well. Add onion powder, black pepper and toss.

5) Take a baking sheet and spray with cooking spray or oil. Pour the mixture over the sheet, place into the oven and bake for 25 minutes.

6) Take the sheet out of the oven and carefully stir the sweet potatoes. Sprinkle with pepper and salt and put the baking sheet into the oven again.

7) In the last 5 minutes of cooking add the garlic to the hash and let it bake for a little bit longer. Check for when the sweet potatoes turn darker, it is OK as it means the potatoes are ready.

8) Serve the hash with scrambled eggs or fresh parsley, add bacon strips if desired.

Bon Appetite!

Grilled Cabbage Steaks with Bacon

The crispy cabbage steaks are great when cooked with a flavorful and spicy marinade. Dress steaks with green fresh onion and crispy bacon and you have yourself a healthy but delicious meal. Adding sweetener to the marinade gives the steaks an unforgettable taste!

Ingredients (7 servings):

6 slices	bacon
1 package	Applewood Marinade
3 tbsp	vegetable oil
2 tbsp	cider vinegar
1 head	green cabbage
2 tablespoons	sweetener
2 tablespoons	green onions

Directions:

1) Take one cabbage, cut it into large slices, about 5-6 steaks.

2) Wash the green onions and slice thinly. Set aside.

3) Slice the bacon into strips.

4) Take a skillet, add vegetable oil to it and put over medium heat. Once the oil begins to simmer, place the bacon strips into the bottom of the skillet. Once the bacon is crumbled, remove it from the heat and set aside.

5) Take a medium-sized bowl, mix oil, vinegar, sweetener, salt, and pepper.

6) Place the cabbage steak into a large bowl, add marinade, cover and refrigerate for about an hour.

7) Once the time is over, remove the cabbage steaks from the marinade, set the marinade aside.

8) Grill the cabbage steaks over the medium heat for 7-9 minutes per each side. Sprinkle with the rest of the marinade from time to time.

9) Serve the cooked cabbage steaks with bacon strips. Dress with green onions.

Bon Appetite!

Cauliflower Soup

This super tender cauliflower soup is amazing for cold winter days. This healthy alternative is unbelievable and flavorful. Try it for yourself!

Ingredients (9 servings):

3 tablespoons	olive oil
1 pound	leeks
2 stalks	celery
3 cloves	garlic
1 large head	cauliflower
2 quarts	chicken or vegetable stock
1 pce	bay leaf
1 teaspoon	sea salt
2 teaspoons	black pepper

chives or thyme for garnish

Directions:

1) Take the pot and heat the olive oil over high heat.

2) Clean and chop the leeks.

3) Dice celery. Peel and mince garlic.

4) Cut cauliflower into 2-3 inch pieces.

5) Add cauliflower, celery, leeks and garlic to the pot. Dress with salt, add pepper. Sauté over low heat. Stir everything well.

6) Add stock and bay leaf to the pot. Cover and cook everything for 30 minutes. Cauliflower must get very tender.

7) Using the food processor blend the soup until smooth.

8) Once blended, place it over medium heat again for 12 minutes.

9) Serve with chopped cilantro.

Bon Appetite!

Salads

Fun Summer Salad

Fresh, green salad full of vitamins and minerals is great for hot summer days. Add your favorite spices to the salad, mix it with vegetable or some other oil or a yoghurt if you wish.

Ingredients (11 servings):

1 head	cauliflower
2 pcs	turnips
4	eggs
2 ribs	celery
¼ cup	minced dill
¼ cup	parsley
2 Tbsp	cider vinegar
1 ½ cups	unsweetened coconut yogurt (A-2 milk)
1 Tbsp	yellow mustard
½ tsp	black pepper
½ tsp	sea salt

Directions:

1) Wash the cauliflower, cut it into medium-sized florets. Cook until tender.

2) Peel the turnips and steam until tender.

3) Boil the eggs and chop them finely.

4) Wash and mince the celery. Wash and chop the dill.

5) Wash the parsley and chop it finely. Set aside.

6) Take a large mixing bowl, combine cauliflower florets, turnips, add chopped eggs, celery, parsley and dill. Toss everything well. Set aside.

7) Take another little bowl, combine vinegar, mustard, a little bit pepper and salt, toss everything well.

8) Pour the dressing over the vegetables and mix well until evenly coated. Add the coconut yoghurt.

Bon Appetite!

Roasted Yam and Kale Salad

This vegetable recipe is super quick, tender and easy. This is the best side dish for roasted meat, grilled fish or seafood. And you don't have to spend a lot of time making it.

Ingredients (6 servings):

2   yams

2 tablespoons   olive oil

salt as desired

black pepper if desired

1 tbsp   olive oil

1 bunch   kale

2 tbsp   red wine vinegar

1 teaspoon   fresh thyme

Directions:

1) Before cooking the dish, preheat the oven to 425 degrees F.

2) Wash the yams. Chop into into 1-inch cubes. Take a little bowl. Mix the yams with olive oil.

3) Sprinkle with salt as desired. Add pepper, place the cubes onto a baking sheet.

4) Bake the yams in the preheated oven until the cubes are tender. It takes around 20 minutes. Let them cool a little bit in the refrigerator.

5) While the yams are cooling, heat the olive oil in a medium-sized skillet. Place it over medium heat. Chop kale into medium-sized pieces.

6) Stir the kale until tender and wilted. Once the kale mix is ready, transfer it to a bowl and put into the refrigerator to cool.

7) Once all of the necessary ingredients are cooled, combine them, add vinegar. Add fresh thyme and toss everything.

8) Sprinkle with pepper if desired, add salt and stir to combine.

Bon Appetite!

Spinach Salad with Bacon-Wrapped Seared Scallops

This delicious spinach salad is amongst my favorites for parties. I cook it all the time as it is so quick and tasty! Serve it over a large plate and dress with parsley or fresh cilantro.

Ingredients (4 servings):

8 pcs   bay scallops

8 pieces   bacon

2 handfuls   baby spinach

1 tsp   coconut oil

Toothpicks

Salt and pepper as desired

Directions:

1) Wash and dry the spinach leaves with a paper towel.

2) Distribute the spinach leaves onto a medium-sized plate.

3) Wash the scallops in cold water. Dry them with a paper towel.

4) Cut bacon in long slices. Set aside.

5) Wrap each of the scallops in a slice of bacon. Fix with the toothpick.

6) Take a little skillet, add coconut oil and fry the bacon-wrapped scallops. It should take you about 2-3 minutes per side. Flip them and fry again.

7) Take a large plate and place the scallops over the spinach bed.

8) Sprinkle with parsley.

Bon Appetite!

"Petit Dejeuner" Salad

This time I would like to offer you an unusual salad recipe with endive greens. Try to surprise your guests with this fresh and light salad. Prepare it for the late supper or for breakfast!

Ingredients:

1/2   endive head

1 egg   poached

2 Tbsp   olive oil

2 strips   bacon chopped

Salt as desired

pepper if desired

Directions:

1) Take a medium-sized skillet, add olive oil and place over medium heat.

2) Chop the bacon strips and put into the skillet once the oil begins to simmer.

3) Fry the bacon strips until tender and crispy. Once the bacon strips are ready, take the strips from the heat.

4) Place the pot with water over the high heat. Place an egg into the water and let it boil for 3 minutes. If you don't like the poached egg, cook it for a little less and remove while the yolk is still runny. In this case, the yolk could be used a part of the dressing.

5) Take the endive head and chop it finely and carefully with the knife.

6) Take a large plate and place the endive green on a plate.

7) Drizzle with olive oil. Put the poached egg over the endive greens. Place the bacon strips over the egg, sprinkle with pepper and salt.

Bon Appetite!

Healthy Tuna Salad in Avocados

Tuna salad served inside of a fresh avocado seems like a delicious and amazing dish! Avoid boring recipes while cooking for your closest family members, lovers, and friends. Surprise them today with these avocadoes!

1 (4.5 oz) cans   Tuna

1   Avocado

1/4 cup   Cilantro leaves

Black pepper as desired

1 tbsp   balsamic

½ cup   cheese cream (from A 2 milk)

1 tsp   Salt

1) Wash the ripe avocado, cut into halves. Take out the seed. Set them aside on a plate.

2) Open the can of tuna carefully and add the tuna into a large mixing bowl.

3) Wash fresh cilantro leaves and dry with a paper towel. Chop them finely.

4) Add chopped cilantro leaves into the bowl with tuna.

5) Sprinkle with balsamic vinegar. Add salt as desired. Sprinkle with black pepper. Mix everything well.

6) Add cream cheese to the mix. Toss everything well once more.

7) Take an avocado half and fill with salad.

8) Serve on a plate. Dress with fresh cilantro leaves as desired.

Bon Appetite!

Chicken Salad with Italian Dressing

This chicken salad with flavorful Italian dressing is amazing and delicious. You only need 8 simple ingredients to cook both the salad and the dressing.

Ingredients (8 servings):

Dressing:

2 cloves	garlic
1/2 cup	avocado oil
1/2 teaspoon	black pepper (as desired)
1 1/2 teaspoon	sea salt (as desired)

Salad:

1/2 head	romaine lettuce
2 cups	chicken
1	avocado chopped
1/2 cup	jicama

Directions:

Dressing:

1) Peel the garlic and mince it finely.

2) Place the garlic into the food processor. Add salt and pepper as desired. Pour the avocado oil.

3) Blend all together.

Salad:

1) Place the pot over medium-high heat. Add water, put the chicken into the water and let it cook for about 20-25 minutes.

2) Once the chicken is ready, remove it from the pot.

3) Let it cool and cut into small pieces. Set aside.

4) Take a medium-sized bowl, add lettuce and chopped chicken.

5) Wash the avocado, peel and slice into small pieces.

6) Cut jicama and add to a mixing bowl.

7) Toss all the ingredients thoroughly. Add salt or pepper to taste.

8) Pour the dressing over the salad.

Bon Appetite!

Conclusion

The most important thing you should remember following the lectin-free diet is that it is almost impossible to completely eliminate lectins from your life. Our main goal is to reduce the consumption of lectins to as low a level as possible. The lectins that are found in grains, nuts, and legumes are something you simply have to avoid if you want to stay healthy. This is the first point I would like to stress. The special lectin-free meal plan shows how to lower the lectin consumption choosing dishes for an entire week. I'm sure that you have already tried a lot of diets searching for the best one and trying to join in on the healthy eating with healthy living. The thing is that many people have never heard of lectins and the harm they cause to a human body. It is hard to imagine living a day without foods you have been eating your entire life. But don't worry this is what this book is for, to offer lectin-free, healthy substitutes for some of your all-time favorites.

 Remember that only a third of all foods you eat every day are high in lectins. The majority of the lectins could be avoided by cooking, fermenting, and sprouting your food. All the foods that are allowed during the lectin-free diet are included in my healthy recipes. These foods have amazing health benefits, are full of minerals and vitamins and what is also important – they could be simply found in the nearest store! And sure, a lot of you may think "I'm healthy now, I don't need some diet or some additional knowledge about lectins and the problems that may cause". Of course, I'm happy if you are 90 years old, full of energy and health. But unfortunately, the majority of us have already been faced with heath issues and the digestive health issues are amongst the most common. Now it is the right time to follow my recommendations and change your life!

Thanks ever so much to each of my cherished readers for investing the time read this book!

I know you could have picked from many other books but you chose this one. So big thanks for downloading this book and reading all way to the end.

If you enjoyed this book or received value from it, I'd like to ask you for a favor. Please take a few minutes to post an honest and heartfelt review on Amazon.com Your support does make a difference and to benefit other people.

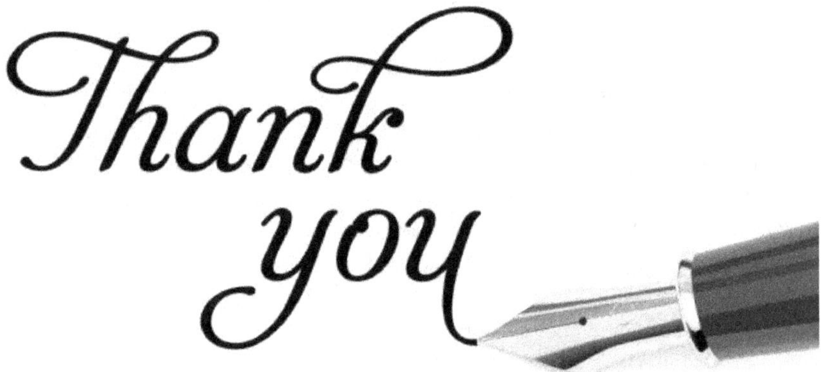